KETOSIS

A 30 Days Easy to Prepare Keto Meal Plan That Turns Your Body Into A Fat Burning Machine

(Lose Up To 10 Pounds in Your First Week)

SANDRA WOODS

Copyright Sandra Woods © 2017

All rights reserved. No part of this publication *Ketosis* may be reproduced, stored in a retrieval system or transmitted in any form or by any means, electronic, mechanical, photocopying, recording, scanning or by any form without permission in writing by the author.

ISBN-13: 978-1983490194

ISBN-10: 1983490199

Contents

Contents

Contents ii

About the Author xiv

Dedication xv

Introduction 1

Day 1 11

Lunch 12

Perfect Bacon Cheeseburger 12

Dinner 13

Low Carb Deep Dish Quiche Pizza 13

Day 2 15

Breakfast 15

Creamy Strawberry Crepes 15

Lunch 16

Ham and Asparagus Brunch Cake 16

Dinner 18

Lemon Marinated Sirloin Steak 18

Day 3 19

Breakfast 19

Lunch 20

German Cucumber Salad (Gurkensalat) 20

Dinner 21

Broccoli Turkey Casserole 21

Day 4 22

Breakfast 22

Roger Verges Fried Eggs with Red Wine Vinegar .. 22

Lunch 23

Quick Salami Roll-Ups 23

Dinner 24

Mexican Veal Sausages 24

Day 5 25

Breakfast 25

Sausage and Egg Muffins 25

Lunch 26

Ham and Cheese Roll 26

Dinner 27

Golden Mushroom and Chicken 27

Lunch 27

Spicy Sausage and Ground Beef Meatballs 27

Day 6 28

Breakfast 28

Dinner 29

Southwest Beef Skillet 29

Day 7 30

Breakfast 30

Zucchini Muffins 30

Lunch 32

Tuna and Avocado Salad 32

Dinner 33

Dill Trout 33

Day 8 34

Breakfast 34

Baked Eggs and Bacon 34

Lunch 35

Shrimp and Nori Rolls 35

Dinner 36

Pinwheel Shepherds Pie 36

Day 9 37

Breakfast 37

Breakfast Burrito 37

Lunch 38

Garlic Mashed Turnips 38

Dinner 39

Crustless Spinach Quiche 39

Day 10 40

Breakfast 40

Spinach and Cheese Omelet 40

Lunch 42

CLASSIC BLT 42

Dinner 43

Filet Mignon with Portobello Sauce 43

Day 11 44

Breakfast 44

Buttery Waffles with Strawberries 44

Lunch 45

Cream Cheese and Turkey Roll Ups w/ Pork Rinds 45

Dinner 46

Mustard-Glazed Halibut Steak 46

Day 12 47

Breakfast 47

Spicy Sausage and Ground Beef Meatballs 47

Dinner 48

Southwestern Skillet 48

Day 13 49

Breakfast 49

Alternative French Toast 49

Lunch 50

Chicken Breast Stir Fry 50

Dinner 51

Ground Beef and Cabbage Casserole 51

Day 14 52

Breakfast 52

Shrimp and Cheese Omelet 52

Lunch 53

Pumpkin and Macadamia Soup 53

Dinner 54

Easy Meatloaf 54

Day 15 55

Breakfast 55

Phony Macaroni and Cheese 55

Lunch 56

Bacon Cheeseburger 56

Dinner 57

Low Carb Deep Dish Quiche Pizza 57

Day 16 59

Breakfast 59

Burger Breakfast Scramble 59

Lunch 60

Spinach Salad with Hot Bacon Dressing 60

Dinner 61

Drunken Chicken 61

Day 17 62

Breakfast 62

Low Carb Cauliflower Hash Browns 62

Lunch 63

Tandoori Chicken Wings 63

Dinner Beef Goulash 64

Day 18 65

Breakfast 65

Upside-down Breakfast Soufflé 65

Lunch 66

Low Carb Chili 66

Dinner 67

Grilled Shrimp and Chicken 67

Day 19 69

Breakfast 69

Fried Eggs with Red Wine Vinegar 69

Lunch 70

Salami Roll Ups 70

Dinner 71

Mexican Veal Sausages 71

Day 20 72

Breakfast 72

Ham and Cheese Breakfast Muffins 72

Lunch 73

Cucumber Tuna Boats 73

Dinner 74

Pork Medallions Dijon 74

Day 21 75

Breakfast 75

Strawberry Crepes 75

Lunch 77

Ham-Asparagus Brunch Cake 77

Dinner 78

Lemon Marinated Sirloin 78

Day 22 79

Breakfast Pizza in a Skillet 79

Lunch 80

Canadian Cheddar Soup 80

Dinner 81

Herb and Garlic Fish 81

Day 23 82

Breakfast 82

Sweet Breakfast Rolls 82

Lunch 84

Garlic Aioli Chicken Wrap 84

Dinner 85

Sesame Beef 85

Day 24 86

Breakfast 86

Egg, Tomato and Parmesan Bake 86

Lunch 87

Egg Drop Chicken Soup 87

Dinner 88

Country Herbed Meatloaf 88

Day 25 90

Breakfast Zucchini Muffins 90

Lunch 91

Tuna and Avocado Salad 91

Dinner 92

Dill Trout 92

Day 26 93

Breakfast Salmon Omelet 93

Lunch 94

Egg Salad over Lettuce 94

Dinner 94

Diet Tuna Casserole 94

Day 27 95

Breakfast 95

Lunch 96

Ham and Cheese Roll 96

Dinner 97

Golden Mushroom Chicken Thighs 97

Day 28 98

Breakfast 98

Mexican Breakfast 98

Lunch 99

Basil Cheese Torta with Red Bell Pepper Strips and Nuts 99

Dinner 100

Beef Baked with Yogurt and Black Pepper 100

Day 29 101

Breakfast 101

Orange Nut Muffins 101

Lunch 103

German Cucumber Salad 103

Dinner 104

Turkey Broccoli Casserole 104

Day 30 105

Breakfast 105

Cinnamon Bran Muffins 105

Lunch 106

Sausage Frittata 106

Dinner 107

Deviled Chicken Halves 107

Conclusion... 109

About the Author

Sandra Woods is a professional chef with 18 years' experience. She is a passionate advocate of ketogenic and anti-aging diets. She emphasis the health benefits of low-carbo lifestyle to women and men alike. Her area of expertise includes recipe development, holistic health, and restricted diets.

She has authored several books including Home-Made Keto smoothies and juices as well as Home Made Italian Pizza. She runs a successful Keto-based pizza spot called pizza place at Sturbridge, Massachusetts, USA.

Dedication

This book is dedicated to all lovers of healthy meals and those who are not satisfied until they learn new ways of preparing one.

"You learn to cook so that you don't have to be a slave to recipes. You get what's in season and you know what to do with it"

- *Julia Child*

Introduction

You may be feeling awful about your weight and physical appearance, but let me tell you this: the moment that you decided that you need to do something about your dilemma (like purchasing this book), means you're already halfway to losing weight, improving your health, and becoming a better version of you. But before I introduce this effective and revolutionary diet that will help solve your problems, let's straighten a few things up. Let me ask you a few fundamental questions that may just shift your perspective:

What is the real reason why you want to shed the fat and lose weight? Is it to boost your confidence and have the perfect bikini body? Or is it so that you can run that marathon you have always wanted to?

You see, nothing wrong with wanting to lose weight to become more attractive, but should this be your focus? This may be your initial goal, but after committing to the Ketogenic lifestyle you will soon realize that the benefits are far more extensive than just mere weight loss.

Mood stabilization, hormone regulation, slowed ageing, blood sugar balance, memory and cognitive improvement. THESE are just a few of the profound changes your body will embrace should you choose to follow the advice that is contained in the pages to follow.

So, besides achieving a "desirable" body, your main purpose will rapidly shift to becoming a healthy, energetic person, avoiding the severe complications of being overweight or obese. Experts have recognized that the primary cause of these conditions is a deadly combination of an unhealthy diet, plus a sedentary lifestyle.

This book contains simple plans I have devised, in the course of my seven years experience on the "Low Carb Diet" to help me out and is based on the induction phase of the Atkins diet, the strictest of his 4 phases. It was designed to help get you started, or back on track should you lose your way. Please come back to this book each time you feel yourself slipping back into your old habits, and it will get you back on track. By personally follow its simple steps, you sure will lose around 25-30 lbs. during its 30-day span.

It is highly recommended that you follow a strong vitamin routine during the entire ketosis 30 days meal plan with emphasis on the following vitamins which are effective metabolic stimulators. Chromiun picolinate, bee pollen/bee propolis, B-1 thiamin, radix ginseng, Gamma oryzanol, lecithin sarasaparilla, inosine.

Entering Ketosis

As you now know, the target of the Ketogenic Diet is to allow your body to enter into ketosis; but the question now is, how?

There are three different types of Ketogenic Diets—the Standard Ketogenic Diet (SKD), Cyclical Ketogenic Diet (CKD), and the Targeted Ketogenic Diet (TKD). The latter two variants of the diet will be ignored due to their complexity. People who have sedentary lifestyles and wish to lose weight through this diet are advised to follow the SKD. This variation recommends limiting the consumpt ion of your carbs to 20-50 grams daily, which means your macronutrients should be made up of 70%-75% fat, 20%-25% protein, and 5%-10% carbs. The number of daily calories you can consume, however, relies on your weight, height, age, and activity. If you're unsure how to do this, you can always consult a keto calculator, which are widely available online.

You might be a little skeptical of the Ketogenic Diet right now, especially if you think that carbs currently make up the biggest portion of your diet. Set aside your assumptions for the duration of this book and approach the next two weeks of your life like an experiment. Trust that if you consume a healthy number of calories and eat foods that are nutrient dense (ex. vegetables, and healthy fat), then you don't have to worry about "dieting" at all! You can safely enter into a state of ketosis when following the prescribed guidelines closely.

I'd like to remind you that unlike any other diets, the Keto Diet needs your complete commitment to the diet in order for you to achieve the state of ketosis. Depending on your body type, activity level, and your diet, you can get into ketosis anywhere from 2 days to a week. For beginners, it is advisable that you use urine ketone sticks (such as Ketostix) to monitor the levels of ketones in your body and ensure that you are in ketosis state. This is a useful tip to help you know whether your body is in ketosis and is burning fat as energy, apart from the other obvious indicators like an increase in energy and lack of appetite.

I must advise you, however, that before anything else, it is a must that you ask for a green light from your health care provider if you are planning to follow the Ketogenic Diet; or any type of diet for that matter. Although this diet is over-all safe, even for kids, you have to let your doctor know about this especially if you have existing health conditions.

Pregnant women or those who are breastfeeding aren't encouraged to try the Ketogenic Diet for weight loss because this may have adverse effects on their baby.

Start your diet with a food diary, record everything you eat, what you were doing at the time, and how you felt. That tells you about yourself, your temptation, the emotional states that encourage you to snack and may help you lose once you see how much you eat. There are quite a few good carb counting software programs on the market today but a simple pad and paper works just as well, but you must keep detailed records, to guarantee your success. Instead of eating the forbidden piece of candy, brush your teeth. If you're about to cheat, allow yourself a treat, but make sure it's a low carb treat. More and more grocers are begriming to carry low carb foods, as the low carb diet's popularity steadily increases. If you happen to live in a small community or rural area, don't fret, there are also tons of great online Low Carb Marts to choose from, my favorite happens to be Netrition.com.

When hunger hits, wait 10 minutes before eating and see if it passes. Set attainable goals. Don't say, "I want to lose 50 pounds." Say, "I want to lose 5 pounds a month." Get enough sleep but not too much. Try to avoid sugar at all costs. Highly sweetened foods tend to make you crave more. When baking, use Splenda, a great tasting sugar substitute that can be found, along with about any other low carb snack, treat and item at Synergy.com Drink six to eight glasses of water a day. Water itself helps cut down on water retention because it acts as a natural diuretic. Taken before meals, it dulls the appetite by giving you that "full feeling." Diet with a buddy. Support groups are important, and caring people can help one another succeed. Start your own, even with just one other person. A great online resource for support is e-Diets.com.

Substitute activity for eating. When the cravings hit, walk around the block. This is especially helpful if you eat out of anger. A good and obvious course of action, would be to begin a workout routine. For warehouse prices on everything from treadmills, to stationary bikes and home gyms, make sure and check out SmoothFitness.com. If the pie on the counter is just too great a temptation and you don't want to throw it away, freeze it. If you're a late-night eater, have a low carb snack, such as some pork rinds or a few cheese curds, before bedtime to cut down on cravings. Keep a glass of water by your bed to quiet the hunger pangs that wake you up in the middle of the night.

If you use food as a reward, establish a new reward system. Buy yourself a nonedible reward. Write down everything you eat -everything - including what you taste when you cook. If you monitor what you eat, you can't go off your diet. Again, the easiest way I have found to track my eating habits and records is with CarbTrack. Weigh yourself once a week at the same time. Your weight fluctuates constantly and you can weigh more at night than you did in the morning, a downer if you stuck to your diet all day. Make dining an event. Eat from your own special plate, on your own special place mat, and borrow the Japanese art of food arranging to make your meal, no matter how normal, look lovely. This is a trick that helps chronic over-eaters and bingers pay attention to their food instead of consuming it unconsciously.

Don't shop when you're hungry. You'll only buy higher carb impulse food. Avoid finger foods that are easy to eat in large amounts. Avoid consuming large quantities of coffee & diet sodas, which are so easy to overdo. And this includes alcoholic beverages. Keep plenty of crunchy foods like raw radishes, cauliflower & broccoli on hand. They're low in carbs, and are very satisfying and filling. Leave something on your plate, even if you are a charter member of the Clean The Plate Club. It's a good sign that you can stop eating when you want to, not just when your plate is empty. Lose weight for yourself, not to please your husband, your parents or your friends.

Make the kitchen off-limits at any time other than mealtime. Always eat at the table, never in front of the TV set or with the radio on. Concentrate on eating every mouthful slowly and savoring each morsel. Chew everything from 10 to 20 times and count! Never skip meals. This is perhaps the most important low carb diet tip at all. If you skip a meal, it signals to your body that it may need to store fat in case the next meal does not come soon. You can lose more weight by eating each low carb meal in the day rather than skipping one, believe it or not.

If you are just beginning the low carb diet, limit your carb intake to the suggested rate of 20 grams a day or less over the first two weeks. After only a few days of doing this, your appetite will decrease dramatically.

Day 1

Breakfast

Low Carb Phony Macaroni and Cheese

Ingridients

1 lb. tofu, firm - well-drained *

2 cups cheddar cheese

2 eggs

¼ cup heavy cream salt and pepper to taste

Onion and garlic - to taste

Nutmeg - to taste

Dry mustard – to taste

Cayenne - to taste

Direction

1. Make sure you use the firmest tofu available for this recipe. You may also want to be generous with the spices and use some extra sharp cheese to liven up the normally bland flavor of tofu.
2. Drain tofu well, making sure to squeeze out all extra moisture, and slice into small pieces (use a French fry cutter or equivalent for consistent sizes).

3. In a separate bowl, mix together eggs, cream and cheese. Stir tofu pieces into mixture and add seasonings as desired. Transfer mixture to a casserole dish or greased pie plate and bake at 375 for 30 - 45 minutes or until golden brown.
4. Yields 4 servings

   [Total Net carbs: 2.6 grams per serving]

Lunch

Perfect Bacon Cheeseburger

Ingridients

1 lb ground beef

1 egg

4 oz. cheddar cheese

4 oz. mozzarella cheese

4 slices bacon

garlic powder, salt and pepper

1. Preheat oven to 350.
2. Precook bacon in conventional oven or microwave. When cooked, crumble bacon and set aside as toppings. In a large skillet,

brown ground beef and drain remaining fat. Mix in egg, cheddar, garlic power, salt and pepper to taste. Transfer to a glass casserole dish and top with mozzarella. Bake for 30-35 minutes. Top with bacon crumbles.

3. Yields 3 servings

   [Total net carbs : 2 grams per serving]

Dinner

Low Carb Deep Dish Quiche Pizza

Ingridients

4 ounces cream cheese

3 eggs

¼ cup parmesan cheese

1/3 cup heavy cream

½ teaspoon oregano

2 cups shredded Italian cheese (mozzarella, romano, parm mix - or your choice)

¼ teaspoon garlic powder

¼ cup tomato sauce

1 cup shredded mozzarella

20 slices pepperoni

1. Preheat oven to 375 degrees.

2. In mixing bowl, beat together the eggs and cream cheese until smooth.
3. Stir in heavy cream, parmesan and spices. Pour 2 cups cheese into a nonstick, 13x9 inch baking pan or equivalent.
4. Add egg mixture on top of cheese and blend together so that cheese is suspended in the mixture and not concentrated at the bottom of the pan.
5. Bake in oven approximately 30 minutes and then briefly remove pan to add on layers of mozzarella and pepperoni. Return to oven for 10 more minutes or until dish is bubbly and brown.
6. Yields 4 servings

[Total Net carbs: 6 grams per serving]

[Total Net carbs for Day 1 based on a single serving per meal: 10.6 grams]

Day 2

Breakfast

Creamy Strawberry Crepes

Ingridients

Butter (enough to fry crepes)

3 large eggs

2/3 cup heavy cream

3 tablespoons Dr. Atkins Bake Mix

4 tablespoons sugar substitute

1/8 teaspoon almond extract

¼ teaspoon vanilla extract

½ teaspoon orange zest grated

Strawberry filling:

2 cups strawberries, washed, hulled and sliced

6 tablespoons Sugar Twin sugar substitute

1. Prepare a heavy, 8-inch skillet or crepe pan with heated butter.
2. Whisk all crepe ingredients together in mixing bowl. Once the butter stops foaming, pour 1/6

crepe mixture into skillet, making sure to cover the bottom evenly.
3. Cook until bottom is browned and top is set. Use a spatula to flip the crepe and brown the other side.
4. Once done, transfer to a paper towel. Repeat this procedure with remaining batter and butter.
5. Next, make your filling by combining strawberries with sugar substitute and spoon about 1mil of mixture on each crepe. Add light whipped cream to taste and garnish with remaining strawberries.
6. Yields 6 servings

[*Total Net carbs: 6.6 grams per serving*]

Lunch

Ham and Asparagus Brunch Cake

Ingredients

2 Tablespoons butter

3 Tablespoons sliced green onion

About ½ pound fresh asparagus, cut (about 1 ½ cups)

6 eggs

1/3 cup heavy cream

1 Teaspoon dried mustard

¼ Teaspoon salt

¼ Teaspoon pepper

2 cups cooked ham, chopped

6 ounces Cheddar cheese, shredded

1. Preheat oven to 350. In a large, heavy skillet, melt butter over medium high heat and cook onions and asparagus for 3 minutes.
2. In a large mixing bowl, stir together eggs, cream and seasonings. Place cooked onions, asparagus and ham into a baking dish and pour egg mixture on top.
3. Bake for 10 -15 minutes and sprinkle cheese on top to taste.
4. Yields 10 servings

[Total Net carbs: 2 grams per serving]

Dinner

Lemon Marinated Sirloin Steak

Ingriedients

1 pound steak, your choice of cuts

1 Teaspoon finely shredded lemon peel

½ cup lemon juice

1/3 cup cooking oil

2 Tablespoons sliced green onion

4 Teaspoons Splenda

1 ½ Teaspoons salt

1 Teaspoon Worcestershire sauce

1 Teaspoon prepared mustard

1/8 Teaspoon pepper

1. If steak has fat around edges, be sure to score them first with a knife. Place the steak into a shallow baking dish.
2. Combine all ingredients to make the lemon marinade and pour over steak.
3. Allow to sit in the refrigerator for at least 4 hours so the marinade has a chance to soak in. Grill steak to your preference on an outdoor

grill, adding leftover over marinade during cooking to maintain tenderness.

4. Yields 6 servings

[Total Net carbs: 2 grams per serving]

[Total Net carbs for Day 2 based on a single serving per meal: 10.6 grams]

Day 3

Breakfast

Ingridients

Orange Nut Muffins

6 eggs, separated

¼ Teaspoon cream of tartar

8 Splenda packets

¼ cup soy flour

¼ cup walnuts, ground

1 Teaspoon orange extract, divided

1 Tablespoon Brown Sugar Twin

4 ounces cream cheese

¼ cup heavy cream

8 Splenda packets

1 Teaspoon orange extract

1. Combine egg whites with cream of tartar and 4 Splenda packets and beat until whites are stiff. Sprinkle on 1 Teaspoon orange extract.
2. In a separate bowl, beat egg yolks together with 4 Splenda packets, and 1 Tablespoon Brown Sugar Twin.
3. Add 1 Teaspoon orange extract. Add a spoonful of egg whites mixture to yolk mixture, stir well, then pour entire yolk mixture into egg whites. Fold in 1 cup soy flour and walnuts.
4. Place mixture into 12 greased muffin cups and bake at 350 for 15 minutes. Reduce oven temperature to 325 and bake for another 15 minutes.
5. Yields 12 servings

    [Total Net carbs: 2.3 grams per serving]

Lunch

German Cucumber Salad (Gurkensalat)

Ingridients

2 cucumbers, thinly sliced

4 green onions, thinly sliced

3 small tomatoes

2 Tablespoons snipped parsley

¼ cup sour cream

¼ Teaspoon mustard

2 Tablespoons minced dill

1 Tablespoon vinegar

1 Tablespoon heavy cream

½ Teaspoon salt

½ Teaspoon pepper

1. Dice and combine cucumbers, onions, tomatoes and parsley.
2. Combine dressing ingredients separately then pour over salad and toss lightly. Chill at least 1 hour before serving.
3. Yields 6 servings

[Total Net carbs: 9 grams per serving]

Dinner

Broccoli Turkey Casserole

Ingridients

2 (10 ounces) packages frozen broccoli

2 cups cooked and diced turkey

1 (10 ounce) can cream of mushroom soup

½ cup heavy cream

½ cup Cheddar cheese, grated

1. Preheat oven to 375.
2. Cook broccoli according to package directions.
3. Layer broccoli in a baking dish and spread turkey on top.
4. Combine soup with cream and pour on top of turkey. Sprinkle on grated cheese. Place in oven and bake for 30 minutes.
5. Yields 8 servings

[Total Net carbs: 7 grams per serving]

[Total Net carbs for Day 3 based on a single serving per meal: 19.3 grams]

Day 4

Breakfast

Roger Verges Fried Eggs with Red Wine Vinegar

Ingridients

1 Tablespoon butter

4 eggs

½ Teaspoon salt

1/8 Teaspoon pepper

1/8 Teaspoon marjoram

2 Teaspoons red wine vinegar

1 Teaspoon parsley

1. Break eggs into skillet over 1 Tablespoon melted butter. Add spices and cook until whites are solid. Place eggs onto serving plates.
2. Melt remaining 1 Tablespoon of butter and heat for two minutes. Stir in red wine vinegar and allow mixture to cook for another minute. Pour over eggs. Garnish with parsley
3. Yields 2 servings

[Total Net carbs: 1 gram per serving]

Lunch

Quick Salami Roll-Ups

Ingridients

5 large slices hard salami

1 Tablespoon cream cheese

2 celery stalks

1. Soften cream cheese in microwave and spread on salami, roll up. Enjoy celery on the side.

2. Yields 1 serving

   [Total Net carbs: 5.9 grams per serving]

Dinner

Mexican Veal Sausages

1 ½ pounds ground veal

2 green onions, finely chopped (1/3 cup)

2 tablespoons fresh cilantro, chopped

2 tablespoons green or red salsa

½ teaspoon ground cumin

½ teaspoon salt

¼ teaspoon freshly ground black pepper

2 tablespoons olive oil

¼ cup green or red salsa for garnish

¼ cup sour cream for garnish

1 lime, cut into slices or wedges, for garnish

1. Combine veal, onion and all spices in mixing bowl and blend together (mash together with bare hands for best results!). Shape mixture into 4 sausage links.
2. Heat oil in a nonstick skillet on high heat and brown sausage 8-10 minutes, turning frequently.

3. Yields 4 servings

   [Total Net carbs: 0.5 grams per serving]

   [Total Net carbs for Day 4 based on a single serving per meal: 7.4 grams]

Day 5

Breakfast

Sausage and Egg Muffins

Ingridients

6 oz Ital. sausage

6 eggs

1/8 cup heavy cream

3 oz cheese

1. Preheat oven to 350. Spray large muffin pans with cooking spray. Cut sausage links and place them 2 to a tin.
2. Mix eggs with cream, salt and pepper. Pour into tins over sausage. Sprinkle with 3 oz cheese, layer on remaining egg mixture and top off with cheese again.
3. Bake for approximately 20 minutes or until eggs are done.

4. Yields 3 servings

   [Total Net carbs: 2.3 grams per serving]

Lunch

Ham and Cheese Roll

8 ounces cream cheese, softened

2 cup Cheddar cheese, shredded

1 Teaspoon grated onions

1 Teaspoon dry mustard

½ Teaspoon paprika

2 ¼ ounces deviled ham

1 Tablespoon parsley flakes

½ cup pecans, chopped Parsley sprigs

1. Combine all ingredients except parsley and pecans. Mix well and chill for at least one hour.
2. Shape mixture into 8 inch rolls and coat with pecans. Garnish with parsley and serve with crackers.
3. Yields 8 servings

   [Total Net carbs: 2 grams per serving]

Dinner

Golden Mushroom and Chicken

6 chicken thighs

1 can golden mushroom soup

1. Remove all skin from thighs and rinse chicken under cold water. Place thighs into a crock pot or slow cooker and pour in mushroom soup.
2. Cook on high for 3-4 hours until meat is tender and fall off the bone.
3. Yields 6 servings

   [Total Net carbs: 4 grams per serving]

   [Total Net carbs: 5.3 grams per serving]

Lunch

Spicy Sausage and Ground Beef Meatballs

[Total Net carbs for Day 5 based on a single serving per meal: 14.3 grams]

Day 6

Breakfast

Ingridients

2 tbs minced onion

½ lb shredded Cheddar cheese

Black pepper to taste

1. This recipe makes approximately 50 meatballs, so you'll want to make it in advance and freeze the remainder to use later for quick meals and snacks.
2. Preheat oven to 350 degrees. Combine all ingredients in a bowl and mix well. Roll into 1-½" balls and place on cookie sheet. Bake 20-25 minutes.
3. Yields approximately 50 servings

   [Total Net carbs: less than 1 gram per serving]

Dinner

Southwest Beef Skillet

2 Tablespoons sliced almonds
1 yellow sweet pepper, cut into bite sized strips
1 fresh jalapeno, seeded and chopped
1 Tablespoon olive oil or cooking oil
4 medium tomatoes, peeled and chopped
1 ½ Teaspoons chili powder
1 Teaspoon ground cumin
1 Teaspoon salt
4 eggs
1 medium ripe avocado, seeded and peeled (optional)

1. Toast almonds over medium high heat 4-5 minutes in large skillet and set aside.
2. Return skillet to heat and add cooking oil. When oil is hot, add sweet pepper and jalapeno and cook until tender. Stir in chili powder, cumin, tomatoes and salt. Bring to a boil Reduce heat, cover and simmer for 5 minutes.
3. Break 1 egg into a measuring cup and carefully

slide it into the tomato mixture. Repeat for each remaining egg. Cover and allow eggs to cook for approximately 5 minutes or until whites are set. Spoon egg and tomato mixture to serving plate and sprinkle with salt and pepper to taste.
4. Add toasted almonds and garnish with avocado slices.
5. Yields 4 servings

   [Total Net carbs: 8 grams per serving]

   [Total Net Carbs for Day 6 based on a single serving per meal: about 14.3 grams]

Day 7

Breakfast

Zucchini Muffins

Ingrideints

1 cup Atkins Bake Mix

1 cup finely ground almonds

1- ½ cups granular sugar substitute

2 Teaspoons cinnamon

1 Teaspoon salt

1 Teaspoon baking soda

1 Teaspoon baking powder

1 cup canola oil

4 eggs

1 medium zucchini, coarsely grated

1 Teaspoon vanilla extract

1. Preheat oven to 350. Whisk together all dry ingredients in a large bowl. Mix wet ingredients, including zucchini together in a medium bowl.
2. Stir wet ingredients into dry mix slowly, blending well. Pour mixture into a greased 8 x 4 loaf pan or greased muffin tins, depending on your preference.
3. Bake for approximately one hour until golden brown and toothpick comes out clean.
4. Yields about 12 servings

[Total Net carbs: 3.5 grams per serving]

Lunch

Tuna and Avocado Salad

Ingridients

2 large hard-boiled eggs
2 Teaspoons hot sauce
1 cup avocado, mashed
½ cup onion, chopped
1 can tuna
2 Tablespoons mayonnaise
2 Tablespoons pickle relish Fresh lemon juice
Salt, to taste

1. Peel eggs and mince with dinner fork.
2. Peel avocado and squeeze lemon juice on it to prevent discoloration. Mash avocado in with egg.
3. Drain tuna and mix into egg/avocado, adding onions, mayonnaise, relish, salt and hot sauce.
4. Stir well and serve over a bed of fresh lettuce.

Dinner

Dill Trout

Ingridients

2 pounds pan-dressed trout (or other small fish), fresh or frozen

1 ½ Teaspoons salt

¼ Teaspoon pepper

½ cup butter or margarine

2 Tablespoons dill weed

3 Tablespoons lemon juice

1. Cut fish lengthwise and spread open to season with salt and pepper.
2. Prepare a fry pan with melted butter and dill weed. Place fish flesh side down and fry 2-3 minutes per side. Once done, remove fish and add lemon juice to butter and dill to create sauce for garnishing.
3. Yields 6 servings

   [Total Net carbs: 1 gram per serving]

   [Total Net carbs for Day 7 based on a single serving per meal: 13.5 grams]

Day 8

Breakfast

Baked Eggs and Bacon

Ingridients

6 slices of bacon

6 eggs

1 non-stick muffin pan

1. For each muffin cup, take one slice of bacon and wrap around 4 fingers to shape it into a circle.
2. Place in muffin cup. Crack egg into the center. Repeat for each serving.
3. Place muffin pan in oven and bake at 350 for about 40 minutes.
4. Yields 6 servings

   [Total Net Carbs: 1 gram per serving]

Lunch

Shrimp and Nori Rolls

Ingridients

1 cup shrimp

1 Tablespoon Mayonnaise

1 thinly sliced green onion

2 sheets Nori

1 cucumber diced and seeded

1 Tablespoon toasted Sesame seeds

1. Drain and rinse shrimp. Combine with Mayonnaise and green onions. Lay Nori on flat surface and spoon on the shrimp and green onion mixture.
2. Sprinkle with cucumber and sesame seeds. Roll tightly and cut into bite size pieces.
3. Yields 4 servings

   [Total Net Carbs: 0.94 grams per serving]

Dinner

Pinwheel Shepherds Pie

Ingridients

1lb. lean ground beef

2 tablespoons onion or garlic salt

8 ounces low carb mushroom soup or sauce mix

1 cup ketchup

1lb. package of frozen, mixed vegetables

1lb Atkin's low carb bake mix or equivalent

1. Pre-heat oven to 375 degrees.
2. Mix low carb bake mix into dough per package instructions and roll flat into a circle roughly the same diameter as your skillet. Cut dough into equal sized triangles and roll each triangle once from base to tip. Set aside.
3. In a non-stick skillet, stir in ground beef and onion salt and cook thoroughly until browned.
4. Stir in mushroom soup/sauce, ketchup and mixed vegetables. Bring mixture to a boil, then

reduce heat to medium and cover and simmer 8 - 10 minutes or until vegetables are tender.
5. Remove skillet from heat and arrange dough triangles on top of mixture with the tips pointing to the center. Place skillet in oven and bake at 375 for approximately 20 minutes or until dough turns golden brown.
6. Yields about 8 servings

[Total Net Carbs: 9 grams per serving]

[Total Net Carbs for Day 8 based on single servings per meal: 10.94 grams]

Day 9

Breakfast

Breakfast Burrito

Ingridienta

¼ cup mushrooms

¼ cup zucchini

1/3 cup tomato

1 clove garlic

2 eggs

dash cayenne pepper dash chili powder
2 Tbsp salsa
2 low carb tortilla shells Mexican
Cheese blend

1. Finely chop the garlic and dice the tomato, zucchini and mushrooms.
2. Pour mixture into eggs and add the pepper and chili powder. Stir until blended. Add mixture to skillet and scramble until done.
3. Place a serving in one low carb tortilla shell, sprinkle with cheese and salsa.
4. Yields 2 servings

[Total Net carbs: 6 gram per serving]

Lunch

Garlic Mashed Turnips

Ingridients

3 cups diced turnip

2 cloves garlic, minced

¼ cup heavy cream

3 T melted butter salt, pepper

1. Boil turnips until tender. Drain and mash turnips as you would for mashed potatoes.
2. Stir in heavy cream, butter, salt, pepper and garlic. Use food processor if you prefer to blend until smooth.

Dinner

Crustless Spinach Quiche

Ingridients

1 cup chopped onion

1 cup sliced fresh mushrooms

1 Tbsp. vegetable oil

1 pkg (10 oz) frozen chopped spinach, thawed

2/3 cup finely chopped ham

5 eggs

3 cups Monterey Jack or Cheddar cheese, shredded

1/8 tsp. pepper

1. Pour 1 Tbsp vegetable oil in a large skillet and sauté the onion and mushrooms until tender.
2. Add in the spinach and ham. Continue to cook and stir mixture until the excess moisture evaporates. Allow to cool slightly.

3. Beat in the eggs and then add cheese, spinach and pepper, making sure to blend well.
4. Spread mixture evenly into a greased 9 inch pie plate or quiche dish and bake at 350 degrees 40-45 minutes or until a knife inserted near the center comes out clean.
5. Yields about 4 servings

[Total Net Carbs: 6 grams per serving]

[Total Net carbs for Day 9 based on single servings per meal : 17 grams].

Day 10

Breakfast

Spinach and Cheese Omelet

Ingridients

Non-stick cooking spray

4 Eggs

Salt

Cayenne Pepper

1 shredded sharp cheddar cheese

1 Tablespoon fresh chives, flat-leaf parsley or chervil

2/3 cup red pepper relish

1. Light coat an eight inch nonstick skillet with cooking spray and heat over medium high heat.
2. In a mixing bowl, beat together the eggs, one dash of salt and one dash of cayenne pepper until mixture is frothy. Pour into skillet. Allow the egg to set, making sure to lift the edges frequently and allow uncooked portion to run under the cooked portion.
3. Continue until egg appears glossy and cooked, but still moist. Add a percentage of the cup of spinach and 2 tablespoons of red pepper relish, topping with cheese and chives.
4. Use spatula to lift-up the edges of the omelet and fold in half.
5. Sprinkle with remaining spinach and red pepper relish. Add additional cheese and chives to taste.

Red Pepper Relish Recipe: 2/3 cup sweet red pepper, 2 Tablespoons chopped onion, 1 Tablespoon cider vinegar, 1 Teaspoon black pepper.

6. Combine all ingredients in a bowl and set aside while preparing omelet. This should make about 2/3 cup of red pepper relish.
7. Yields 1 serving

   [Total Net Carbs : 1 gram per serving]

Lunch

Classsic BLT

Ingridients

4 slices bacon

1 lg. Leaf lettuce

½ sliced tomato mayo

1. In place of bread, you'll be using the lettuce to roll this up. Spread desired amount of Mayonnaise on lettuce, add bacon slices, roll up and enjoy!
2. Yields 1 serving

   [Total Net Carbs: 4.9 grams per serving]

Dinner

Filet Mignon with Portobello Sauce

4 beef tenderloin steaks

1 Teaspoon olive oil

1 Teaspoon black pepper

2 large Portobello mushrooms (halved and sliced)

8 green onions cut into 1 inch pieces

1 Tablespoon butter

1/3 cup reduced sodium beef broth

2 Tablespoons Madeira or Port wine

1. Mix oil with pepper and use to baste both sides of steaks.
2. Prepare sauce in a large skillet as follows: heat butter over medium high heat and sauté mushrooms and onions until tender. Add broth and wine and bring to a boil. Remove from heat.
3. Charcoal grill method for steaks: Grill steaks uncovered over medium hot coals to desired doneness. Turn steaks once halfway through grilling.

4. When done, slice thin and smother with mushroom and onion sauté.
5. Yields 4 servings

   [Total Net Carbs: 3 grams per serving]

   [Total Net carbs for Day 10 based on single servings per meal: 8.9 grams]

Day 11

Breakfast

Buttery Waffles with Strawberries

4 eggs

1 Tablespoon "Just Whites" (egg white powder or substitute)

1 cup cottage cheese

1 Tablespoon gluten flour

2 Tablespoons butter

2 Tablespoons oat bran

1 Teaspoon vanilla extract

1 Teaspoon cream of tartar

1 cup sliced stawberries

1. Mix egg whites from separated eggs with cream of tartar and beat until stiff peaks form.

2. Blend egg yolks, "Just Whites", cottage cheese, gluten flour, butter, oat bran and vanilla separately in a blender until smooth. Fold blended mixture gently into egg whites.
3. Cook with a standard waffle iron coated with a nonstick cooking spray.
4. Yields about 8 servings

   [Total Net carbs: 5.56 grams per serving]

   [single waffle contains 2.25 grams and 1cup strawberries adds 2.91 grams]

Lunch

Cream Cheese and Turkey Roll Ups w/ Pork Rinds

Ingridients

4 slices turkey breast deli meat

4 Tablespoons cream cheese

1 serving pork rinds

1. Put 1 Tablespoon cream heese onto turkey breasts and roll up.
2. Place in microwave for about 20 seconds until cream cheese melts. Enjoy pork rinds on the side.

3. Yield: n/a

   [Total Net carbs: approximately 1.6 grams]

Dinner

Mustard-Glazed Halibut Steak

Ingredients

16 ounce fresh or frozen halibut steak

1 Tablespoon butter

1 Tablespoon lemon juice

1 Tablespoon Dijon mustard

1 Teaspoon fresh basil

1. Fish should be thawed before beginning. Heat butter, basil, lemon juice and mustard in a small saucepan until butter is melted. Brush both sides of halibut steak with mixture.
2. Grill fish over medium hot coals on an outdoor barbecue grill for 8 -12 minutes or until fish begins to flake.
3. Yields 1 serving

   [Total Net carbs; 1 gram per serving]

   [Total Net carbs for Day 11 based on a single serving per meal: 8.16 grams]

Day 12

Breakfast

Spicy Sausage and Ground Beef Meatballs

Ingridients

2 lbs ausage

1 lb ground beef

3 eggs

2 tbs minced onion

½ lb shredded Cheddar cheese black pepper to taste

1. This recipe makes approximately 50 meatballs, so you'll want to make it in advance and freeze the remainder to use later for quick meals and snacks.
2. Preheat oven to 350 degrees. Combine all ingredients in a bowl and mix well. Roll into 1-½ inch balls and place on cookie sheet. Bake 20-25 minutes.
3. Yields approximately 50 servings

   [Total Net carbs: less than 1 gram per serving]

Dinner

Southwestern Skillet

Ingridients

2 Tablespoons sliced almonds

1 yellow sweet pepper, cut into bite sized strips

1 fresh jalapeno, seeded and chopped

1 Tablespoon olive oil or cooking oil

4 medium tomatoes, peeled and chopped

½ Teaspoons chili powder

1 Teaspoon ground cumin

1 Teaspoon salt

4 eggs

1 medium ripe avocado, seeded and peeled (optional)

1. Toast almonds over medium high heat 4-5 minutes in large skillet and set aside. Return skillet to heat and add cooking oil. When oil is hot, add sweet pepper and jalapeno and cook until tender.
2. Stir in chili powder, cumin, tomatoes and salt.
3. Bring to a boil Reduce heat, cover and simmer for 5 minutes. Break 1 egg into a measuring cup and carefully slide it into the tomato

mixture. Repeat for each remaining egg. Cover and allow eggs to cook for approximately 5 minutes or until whites are set. Spoon egg and tomato mixture to serving plate and sprinkle with salt and pepper to taste.
4. Add toasted almonds and garnish with avocado slices.
5. Yields 4 servings

[Total Net carbs: 8 grams per serving]

[Total Net Carbs for Day 12 based on a single serving per meal: about 14.3 grams]

Day 13

Breakfast

Alternative French Toast

Ingridients

2 Eggs

1 cup of heavy whipping cream

2 packages of sugar substitute Cinnamon to taste

1 of a 3 oz. bag of unflavored Pork rinds

1. Crush the pork rinds as finely as you can without turning them into a powder.
2. Mix together the eggs, cream, sweetener and cinnamon and pour into bowl with pork rinds.
3. Stir and allow mixture to soak until you have a thick, goopy batter. Pour in batter and fry pancake style in butter, browning both sides until done.
4. Serve with your favorite low carb syrup.
5. Yields about 2 servings

[Total Net carbs: less than 2 grams per serving]

Lunch

Chicken Breast Stir Fry

Ingridients

1 cup lettuce

1 tomato

1 chopped pepper

1 tbs olive oil

1 chicken breast

A few ounces of your favorite low carb dressing

1. Clean and chop vegetables and slice chicken into stir fry sized pieces.
2. Heat with a little bit of cooking oil and stir fry chicken. When chicken is done, toss into a plastic container with the fresh vegetables and pour in dressing. Close with lid and shake to coat.
3. Yields 1 serving

   [Total Net Carbs: 4 grams per serving]

Dinner

Ground Beef and Cabbage Casserole

Ingridients

1 lb ground beef

1 cup chopped onion

1 bag cole slaw mix

1- ½ cups tomato sauce

2 Tablespoons lemon juice

1. Brown ground beef first and set aside.
2. Add onion and cabbage to skillet and sauté until soft.

3. Add ground beef back in along with tomato sauce and lemon juice.
4. Bring mixture to a boil, then cover and simmer for 30 minutes.
5. Yields 3 servings

   [Total Net carbs: 8 grams per serving]

   [Total Net carbs for Day 13 based on a single serving per meal: about 12 grams]

Day 14

Breakfast

Shrimp and Cheese Omelet

Ingridients

3 medium Eggs

1 tbsp Butter

3 oz Shrimp, chopped

1 oz Shredded Harvarti Cheese, (or Monterey Jack Cheese)

2 tsp Fresh parsley, chopped Green onions, (optional)

1 tsp Basil, chopped (optional)

1. Whisk eggs in bowl with parsley. Transfer to skillet and cook omelet style, adding shrimp, cheese and onions before folding.

2. Top with basil and extra cheese if desired.
3. Yields 1 serving

[Total Net carbs: about 2.72 grams per serving]

Lunch

Pumpkin and Macadamia Soup

Ingridients

1 tablespoon macadamia or olive oil
½ cup roughly chopped macadamias
1 small onion, chopped
1 teaspoon grated ginger
3 cups diced or canned pumpkin
1 small tart apple, chopped
3 cups chicken stock sour cream for topping
Whole or halved macadamias, roasted for garnish

1. Heat oil in a heavy stock pot and sauté macadamias, onions and ginger for 2 minutes.
2. Stir in apple and pumpkin slices and sauté for 2 - 3 minutes (if substituting canned pumpkin puree, add only the apple in the step above and use pumpkin puree when you add chicken stock). Pour in chicken stock. Bring to a boil

then cover and simmer for 20 minutes or until apples/pumpkin become soft. Transfer to blender and blend until smooth.
3. Yields 6 servings

[Total Net carbs: 7.5 grams per serving]

Dinner

Easy Meatloaf

Ingridients

½ lbs ground beef 1 cup pork rind crumbs

1 egg

1/3 cup tomato sauce

2 Tablespoons parsley

1 cup grated parmesan

1 cup chopped onion salt and pepper to taste

1. Mix all ingredients together in a bowl, making sure to distribute pork rind crumbs evenly.
2. Shape mixture into a loaf and place in a shallow nonstick baking pan.
3. Bake in a preheated oven at 350 degrees for 1 hour.
4. Yields 6 servings

[Total Net carbs: 1.8 grams per serving]

[Total Net carbs for Day 14 based on a single serving per meal: 12.02 grams]

Day 15

Breakfast

Phony Macaroni and Cheese

1 lb. tofu, firm - well-drained *

2 cups cheddar cheese

2 eggs

¼ cup heavy cream

salt and pepper - to taste

onion and garlic - to taste

nutmeg - to taste

dry mustard - to taste

cayenne - to taste

*Make sure you use the firmest tofu available for this recipe. You may also want to be generous with the spices and use some extra sharp cheese to liven up the normally bland flavor of tofu.

1. Drain tofu well, making sure to squeeze out all extra moisture, and slice into small pieces (use

a French fry cutter or equivalent for consistent sizes). In a separate bowl, mix together eggs, cream and cheese.
2. Stir tofu pieces into mixture and add seasonings as desired. Transfer mixture to a casserole dish or greased pie plate and bake at 375 for 30 - 45 minutes or until golden brown.
3. Yields 4 servings

[Total Net carbs: 2.6 grams per serving]

Lunch

Bacon Cheeseburger

Ingridients

1 lb ground beef

1 egg

4 oz. cheddar cheese

4 oz. mozzarella cheese

4 slices bacon

garlic powder, salt and pepper

1. Preheat oven to 350.
2. Precook bacon in conventional oven or microwave.

3. When cooked, crumble bacon and set aside as toppings. In a large skillet, brown ground beef and drain remaining fat. Mix in egg, cheddar, garlic power, salt and pepper to taste. Transfer to a glass casserole dish and top with mozzarella. Bake for 30-35 minutes. Top with bacon crumbles.
4. Yields 3 servings

   [Total net carbs : 2 grams per serving]

Dinner

Low Carb Deep Dish Quiche Pizza

4 ounces cream cheese

3 eggs

¼ cup parmesan cheese

1/3 cup heavy cream

½ teaspoon oregano

2 cups shredded Italian cheese (mozzarella, romano, parm mix - or your choice)

¼ teaspoon garlic powder

¼ cup tomato sauce

1 cup shredded mozzarella

20 slices pepperoni

1. Preheat oven to 375 degrees. In mixing bowl, beat together the eggs and cream cheese until smooth. Stir in heavy cream, parmesan and spices.
2. Pour 2 cups cheese into a nonstick, 13x9 inch baking pan or equivalent. Add egg mixture on top of cheese and blend together so that cheese is suspended in the mixture and not concentrated at the bottom of the pan.
3. Bake in oven approximately 30 minutes and then briefly remove pan to add on layers of mozzarella and pepperoni. Return to oven for 10 more minutes or until dish is bubbly and brown.
4. Yields 4 servings

   [Total Net carbs: 6 grams per serving]

   [Total Net carbs for Day 15 based on a single serving per meal: 10.6 grams]

Day 16

Breakfast

Burger Breakfast Scramble

Ingridients
1 lb ground beef
2 Tablespoons minced onion
3 oz cream cheese
3 large eggs
1 Tablespoon water salt, pepper

1. Ground beef and onions together in a skillet.
2. Add cream cheese and cook over low heat until melted. Beat together the eggs, water, salt and pepper and pour into skillet.
3. Scramble until done.
4. Yields 2 servings

[Total Net carbs: 2.11 grams per serving]

Lunch

Spinach Salad with Hot Bacon Dressing

1 bag fresh baby spinach
¼ chopped onion
4 slices bacon
2 hard boiled eggs, chopped
¼ cup vinegar
1 pkg Splenda salt, pepper

1. Cook bacon and allow to drain on paper towel, but keep bacon grease in pan. Add vinegar, pepper and Splenda to bacon grease. Stir and heat slowly until boiling. Tear spinach into salad sized pieces and toss with toss egg, onion and crumbled bacon.
2. Immediately pour on hot dressing and toss lightly.
3. Yields 2 servings

   [Total Net carbs: 5 grams per serving]

Dinner

Drunken Chicken

Ingridients

4 boneless skinless chicken breasts OR
4 split fryer breasts - skinned.
1 Tablespoons Butter
½ small onion, minced
1 clove garlic, crushed
1 Tablespoon parsley
1 Tablespoon Brown Sugar Twin
1 Tablespoon mustard
½ cup chicken stock
¼ cup red wine
4 Tablespoons Gin

1. Preheat oven to 350 degrees. In a large skillet, sauté the butter and chicken until chicken is browned. Remove chicken and set aside.
2. Add onion to skillet and sauté until soft.
3. Puree remaining ingredients in a blender the add to skillet and heat through. Place chicken in a baking dish and pour mixture on top. Bake 15 -20 minutes for boneless breasts.

4. Bake 30-40 minutes for bone in split breasts.
5. Yields 4 servings

   [Total Net carbs: less than 1 gram per serving]

   [Total Net carbs for Day 16 based on a single serving per meal: about 8.11 grams]

Day 17

Breakfast

Low Carb Cauliflower Hash Browns

Ingridients

12 oz grated fresh cauliflower (about V2 medium head)

4 slices bacon - chopped

3 oz. chopped onion

1 Tablespoon butter, softened salt, pepper

1. Sauté bacon and onion in skillet just until brown. Add in cauliflower and stir until tender and browned all over, adding butter throughout cooking. Season to taste with salt and pepper.
2. Yields 2 servings

   [Total Net carbs: about 8 grams per serving]

Lunch

Tandoori Chicken Wings

Ingridients

2- ½ lbs chicken wings, trimmed and separated
1 cup Homemade Yogurt
2 Tablespoons ginger
6 cloves garlic, minced
1 Teaspoons curry powder
1 Teaspoon turmeric
1 Teaspoon cumin
1 Teaspoon dry mustard
2 Teaspoons red pepper flakes
1 lemon, juiced
3 Tablespoons vegetable oil salt, pepper

1. Mix all ingredients in a bowl. Marinade for at least two hours at room temperature.
2. Saving marinade, put wings on broiling rack and broil until browned and cooked through, (about 20 minutes) basting wings with marinade about every 10 minutes.
3. Transfer to platter and serve.

4. Mix milk and cream together and boil in a saucepan. Remove from heat and allow to cool to room temperature. Stir in yogurt. Cover and keep in a warm place for approximately 20-30 hours.
5. Yields 4 servings

   [Total Net carbs: 4 g rams per serving]

Dinner Beef Goulash

Ingridients

2 lbs beef cubed, in 1- ½ inch cubes

3 Tablespoons cooking oil

1 Tablespoon chili salsa

3 oz onions, chopped

1 sweet bell pepper, cubed

1 lb tomatoes, cubed

1 cup red wine

water

salt, pepper

1. Fry cubed beef in a large pot or skillet in cooking oil. Once beef browns, add chili salsa

and fry for 1 minute. Add onions and cubed vegetables and continue frying for 10 minutes.
2. Add wine as well as extra water if needed. Cover and simmer for 30 minutes. Add salt and pepper to taste.
3. Yields 4 servings

[Total Net carbs: 5.5 grams per serving]

[Total Net carbs for Day 17 based on a single serving per meal: 17.5 grams]

Day 18

Breakfast

Upside-down Breakfast Soufflé

½ cup egg whites

3 Tablespoons unsalted butter

1 cup thinly sliced mushrooms

1 medium tomato, thinly sliced

salt and pepper to taste

1 cup crumbled fresh goat cheese, or cheese of your choice

1. Preheat oven to 400 degrees. Add salt and pepper to egg whites and whip into soft peaks.

2. In a heavy, oven safe frying pan or cast iron skillet, heat the butter over high heat and sauté mushrooms until soft. Place tomato slices over mushroom.
3. Quickly fold cheese into egg white mixture and pour on top of mushroom/tomato mixture. Place pan in oven and bake for approximately 8 minutes. Remove from oven and flip soufflé over onto serving plate.
4. Yields 1 serving

[Total Net carbs: 6 grams per serving]

Lunch

Low Carb Chili

Ingridients

2 cloves minced garlic

1 cup chopped onions

3 Tablespoons olive oil

2 lbs lean beef, chopped

4 cups canned tomatoes, drained or 4 cups beef both 2 Teaspoons salt (omit if using broth)

2 bay leaves

1 Teaspoon oregano

1 Teaspoon crushed cumin

2-3 Tablespoons chili powder

2 cans Eden Black soybeans, drained

1. Place all ingredients in a large stock pot or slow cooker. Bring to a boil. Reduce heat, cover and simmer for 1- 2 hours. The longer this mix simmers, the more the flavors will set in. For extra carb reduction: substitute beef broth or stock in place of tomatoes (broth version reduces carbs to 3.2 grams per serving).
2. Yields 12 servings

[Total Net carbs: 8.5 grams per serving]

Dinner

Grilled Shrimp and Chicken

Ingridients

1/4 teaspoon poultry seasoning

1/8 to 1/4 teaspoon cayenne pepper

1/8 teaspoon white pepper

1/8 teaspoon onion powder

1 tablespoon garlic powder

2 tablespoons butter

½ pint heavy cream

½ cup chicken broth

1 tablespoon olive oil

½ cup white wine

4 skinless, boneless chicken breasts

8 ounces shrimp

Grated Romano cheese for garnish

1. Combine the poultry seasoning, cayenne pepper, white pepper, onion powder and garlic powder in a small bowl, then divide in half.
2. Melt butter in skillet over low heat and add cream, broth and 1 spice mixture. Stir well and allow to thicken into sauce. Set aside.
3. Preheat grill to high heat.
4. Heat cooking oil over medium high heat in a large skillet. Add chicken breasts and sauté with remaining spice mixture until chicken is cooked through. Remove from heat and set aside.
5. Lightly oil grill grates. Place shrimp on hot grill and cook for 3 to 4 minutes or until cooked through. Serve each chicken breast topped

with grilled shrimp and covered with cream sauce. Garnish with Romano cheese.

6. Yields 4 servings

[Total Net carbs: 3 grams per serving]

[Total Net carbs for Day 18 based on a single serving per meal: 17.5 grams]

Day 19

Breakfast

Fried Eggs with Red Wine Vinegar

Ingridients

1 Tablespoon butter

4 eggs

1 Teaspoon salt

1/8 Teaspoon pepper

1/8 Teaspoon marjoram

2 Teaspoons red wine vinegar

1 Teaspoon parsley

1. Break eggs into skillet over 1 Tablespoon of melted butter. Add spices and cook until whites are solid. Place eggs onto serving

plates. Melt remaining 1 Tablespoon of butter and heat for two minutes.
2. Stir in red wine vinegar and allow mixture to cook for another minute. Pour over eggs. Garnish with parsley
3. Yields 2 servings

   [Total Net carbs: 1 gram per serving]

Lunch

Salami Roll Ups

Ingridients

5 large slices hard salami

1 Tablespoon cream cheese

2 celery stalks

1. Soften cream cheese in microwave and spread on salami, roll up. Enjoy celery on the side.
2. Yields 1 serving

   [Total Net carbs: 5.9 grams per serving]

Dinner

Mexican Veal Sausages

1 ½ pounds ground veal
2 green onions, finely chopped (1/3 cup)
2 tablespoons fresh cilantro, chopped
2 tablespoons green or red salsa
½ teaspoon ground cumin
½ teaspoon salt
¼ teaspoon freshly ground black pepper
2 tablespoons olive oil
¼ cup green or red salsa for garnish
¼ cup sour cream for garnish
1 lime, cut into slices or wedges, for garnish

1. Combine veal, onion and all spices in mixing bowl and blend together (mash together with bare hands for best results!). Shape mixture into 4 sausage links. Heat oil in a nonstick skillet on high heat and brown sausage 8-10 minutes, turning frequently.
2. Yields 4 servings

[Total Net carbs: 0.5 grams per serving]

[Total Net carbs for Day 19 based on a single serving per meal: 7.4 grams]

Day 20

Breakfast

Ham and Cheese Breakfast Muffins

Ingridients

6 large eggs, separated
1 teaspoon cream of tartar
½ cup cottage cheese
¼ cup Dr. Atkins Bake Mix
1 teaspoon salt
2 tablespoons green onion, minced
2 tablespoons butter, melted
1 teaspoon Sugar Twin sugar substitute
2 cups ham
1 cup cheddar cheese, cubed
½ cup cream

1. Place separated egg whites into a mixing bowl along with the cream of tartar and set aside. Place egg yolks in another bowl and add remaining ingredients one by one, making sure

to stir after each addition. Whip eggs whites and cream of tartar until still, then fold into egg yolk mixture.
2. Pour mixture evenly into nonstick, buttered muffin pans and bake at 350 degrees for 30 - 35 minutes.
3. Yields 16 servings

   [Total Net carbs: 1 gram per serving]

Lunch

Cucumber Tuna Boats

3 cucumbers

1 can tuna

2 hard boiled eggs, diced

½ cup Cheddar cheese, shredded

½ cup celery, diced

¼ cup mayonnaise

2 Tablespoons dill relish

1 Tablespoon chopped onion

1 Teaspoon lemon juice

½ Teaspoon salt

1. Cut cucumbers lengthwise and de-seed. Cut a small slice off the bottom to make cucumbers lay flat.
2. Combine remaining ingredients in mixing bowl to make tuna salad and spoon into cucumbers. Serve immediately.
3. Yields 6 servings

   [Total Net carbs: 5 grams per serving]

Dinner

Pork Medallions Dijon

Ingridients

2 lbs pork tenderloins cut into

1 inch thick rounds

2 Tablespoons butter or olive oil

1 cup sliced shallots

4 Tablespoons heavy cream

1/3 cup chicken broth

3 Tablespoons capers, drained

2 Tablespoons coarse Dijon mustard

1. Flatten pork rounds to 6 inch thickness and season with salt and pepper to taste.

2. Heat butter or olive oil in skillet and sauté tenderloin rounds approximately 2 minutes per side or until browned.
3. Transfer to plate. Add in shallots and sauté for 1 minute. Add sauce and heavy cream and proceed to boil until sauce thickens enough to coat a spoon.
4. Mix in capers and mustard, and return tenderloins to sauce in skillet to heat through.
5. Yields 4 servings

[Total Net carbs: 4 grams per serving]

[Total Net carbs for Day 20 based on a single serving per meal : 10 grams]

Day 21

Breakfast

Strawberry Crepes

Ingridients

Butter (enough to fry crepes)

3 large eggs

2/3 cup heavy cream

3 tablespoons Dr. Atkins Bake Mix

4 tablespoons sugar substitute

1/8 teaspoon almond extract

¼ teaspoon vanilla extract

½ teaspoon orange

zest grated

Strawberry filling:

2 cups strawberries, washed, hulled and sliced

6 tablespoons Sugar Twin sugar

1. Prepare a heavy, 8 inch skillet or crepe pan with heated butter.
2. Whisk all crepe ingredients together in mixing bowl. Once the butter stops foaming, pour 1/6 crepe mixture into skillet, making sure to cover the bottom evenly.
3. Cook until bottom is browned and top is set. Use a spatula to flip the crepe and brown the other side. Once done, transfer to a paper towel. Repeat this procedure with remaining batter and butter.
4. Next, make your filling by combining strawberries with sugar substitute and 1 spoon of mixture on each crepe. Add light whipped

cream to taste and garnish with remaining strawberries.
5. Yields 6 servings

[Total Net carbs: 6.6 grams per serving]

Lunch

Ham-Asparagus Brunch Cake

Ingridients

2 Tablespoons butter

3 Tablespoons sliced green onion

About ½ pound fresh asparagus, cut (about 1 ½ cups)

6 eggs

1/3 cup heavy cream

1 Teaspoon dried mustard

¼ Teaspoon salt

¼ Teaspoon pepper

2 cups cooked ham, chopped

6 ounces Cheddar cheese, shredded

1. Preheat oven to 350. In a large, heavy skillet, melt butter over medium high heat and cook onions and asparagus for 3 minutes.

2. In a large mixing bowl, stir together eggs, cream and seasonings. Place cooked onions, asparagus and ham into a baking dish and pour egg mixture on top. Bake for 10 -15 minutes and sprinkle cheese on top to taste.
3. Yields 10 servings

   [Total Net carbs: 2 grams per serving]

Dinner

Lemon Marinated Sirloin

Ingridients

1 pound steak, your choice of cuts

1 Teaspoon finely shredded lemon peel

½ cup lemon juice

1/3 cup cooking oil

2 Tablespoons sliced green onion

4 Teaspoons Splenda

1 ½ Teaspoons salt

1 Teaspoon Worcestershire sauce

1 Teaspoon prepared mustard

1/8 Teaspoon pepper

1. If steak has fat around edges, be sure to score them first with a knife.

2. Place the steak into a shallow baking dish.
3. Combine all ingredients to make the lemon marinade and pour over steak.
4. Allow to sit in the refrigerator for at least 4 hours so the marinade has a chance to soak in.
5. Grill steak to your preference on an outdoor grill, adding leftover over marinade during cooking to maintain tenderness.
6. Yields 6 servings

[Total Net carbs: 2 grams per serving]

[Total Net carbs for Day 21 based on a single serving per meal: 10.6 grams]

Day 22

Breakfast Pizza in a Skillet

Ingridients

1 egg

2 Tablespoons spaghetti sauce

2 slices Canadian bacon or preferred meat

1 cup sliced black olives

2 oz shredded mozzarella cheese

1 Tablespoon oil

1. Heat oil in a nonstick skillet. Beat eggs and pour into skillet, coating bottom evenly.
2. Flip halfway through cooking when bottom is set. Add spaghetti sauce, meat, olives and cheese. Cook until cheese is melted.
3. Yields 1 serving

   [Total Net carbs: 8 grams per serving]

Lunch

Canadian Cheddar Soup

Ingridients

2 Tablespoons butter

¼ cup onion, chopped

¼ cup chopped celery

2 Tablespoons soy flour

¼ Teaspoon dry mustard

1 pinch nutmeg

1 pinch pepper

3 cups chicken stock

1 ½ cups heavy cream

1 cup water

1 ½ cups Cheddar cheese, shredded

1 dash Worcestershire sauce

1. Melt butter in a heavy sauce pan. Cook onions and celery until tender. Add flour, mustard, nutmeg and pepper and stir, cooking for 2 - 3 minutes.
2. Add chicken stock and simmer for about 20 minutes, stirring occasionally. You may want to use a hand blender to puree the mixture when done. Return soup to stove, adding cream and water and bring close to boiling. Immediately stir in cheese and allow to melt.
3. Add dashes of salt, pepper and Worcestershire sauce to taste.
4. Yields 6 servings

   [Total Net carbs: 6 grams per serving]

Dinner

Herb and Garlic Fish

Ingridients

½ cup mayonnaise

½ Teaspoon dried marjoram leaves

½ Teaspoon dried thyme leaves

½ Teaspoon garlic powder

¼ Teaspoon ground celery seed

1 pound fish fillets

1. Mix dressing and seasonings together and brush mixture on one side of fish.
2. Place fish in a broiler pan on rack in oven 2-4 inches from heat. Broil 5-8 minutes. Turn fish over and coat with remaining mixture and broil for another 5-8 minutes.
3. Yields 4 servings

[Total Net carbs: 1 gram per serving]

[Total Net carbs for Day 22 based on a single serving per meal: 11 grams]

Day 23

Breakfast

Sweet Breakfast Rolls

Ingridients

5 eggs

2 Tablespoons Atkins pancake mix

2 Tablespoons heavy cream

1 package sugar substitute

1 Teaspoon cinnamon

1 Teaspoon vanilla extract

Filling

4 oz cream cheese

1 Teaspoon cinnamon

1 package sugar substitute

1. To make the filling, soften cream cheese in microwave and mix with sugar substitute and cinnamon. Beat eggs with cream and slowly stir in pancake mix, sugar substitute, vanilla extract and cinnamon.
2. Bring a buttered, nonstick skillet to medium high heat and pour in pancake mixture. Cook until done on both sides. Repeat process to make 4 thin pancakes. Spread filling on one side of pancake and roll up to eat.
3. Yields 4 servings

[Total Net carbs: 4.3 grams per serving]

Lunch

Garlic Aioli Chicken Wrap

Ingridients

3 oz canned or vacuum-packed chicken, drained

1 Mission Low Carb Tortilla Garlic

*aioli spread**

Prepare aioli recipe and use as a spread on your low carb tortillia with chicken.

This recipe makes 10 servings of aioli, so you may want save some for dipping.

Garlic Aioli

6 garlic cloves, peeled and halved

1 egg yolk

1 cup extra virgin olive oil

2 Tablespoons lemon juice

1. Mash garlic with a mortar and pestle or use a garlic press. Stir in salt and egg yolk and beat mixture until egg turn a light color.
2. Slowly drizzle in the olive oil, followed by the lemon juice. Stir well and season to taste.
3. Yields 1 serving

[Total Net carbs: 5 grams per serving]

Dinner

Sesame Beef

Ingridients

1 pound sirloin steak, cut into 1/8-inch strips

2 Splenda packets

3 Tablespoons cooking oil, divided

2 Tablespoons soy sauce

¼ Teaspoon pepper

3 green onions, thinly sliced

2 garlic cloves, minced

1 Tablespoon sesame seeds

1. Place beef in a glass bowl. Mix sugar, oil, soy sauce, seasonings and sesame seeds.
2. Pour mixture over beef and toss to coat. Allow to marinate for 15 minutes.
3. Stir fry marinated beef in skillet or wok over high heat.

[Total Net carbs: 2 grams per serving]

[Total Net carbs for Day 23 based on a single serving per meal: 11.3 grams]

Day 24

Breakfast

Egg, Tomato and Parmesan Bake

Ingridients

5 eggs

3 Tablespoons chunky tomato sauce

2 Tablespoons heavy cream

2 Tablespoons grated parmesan cheese

1. Preheat oven to 350. Combine eggs and cream in mixing bowl. Stir in tomato sauce and add the cheese.
2. Pour into a glass baking dish and bake for 25 - 35 minutes. Check cooking progress every 5 minutes after the first 25 minutes have passed to make sure the mixture doesn't burn. The bake is done when a toothpick inserted in the middle comes out clean. Top off with extra cheese and allow to melt.
3. Yields 1 serving

   [Total Net carbs: 7 grams per serving]

Lunch

Egg Drop Chicken Soup

Ingridients

5 cups chicken stock

2 tablespoons soy sauce

2 eggs, well beaten

1. Bring soy sauce and chicken stock to a boil.
2. Beat eggs and pour into boiling soup slowly, from a height of at least 10 inches, stirring quickly with other hand. Once the last of the egg is stirred in, allow to cook for 30 seconds and then remove from heat immediately.
   *Serve with your choice of garnishes. Complementary garnishes include sautéed mushroom, chives or dill.
3. Yields 4 servings
   [Total Net carbs: 2 grams per serving]

Dinner

Country Herbed Meatloaf

Ingridients

Herb Sauce

¼ cup olive oil

8 ounces fresh mushrooms, chopped

1 large onion, finely chopped

1 garlic clove, minced

1 (28 ounce) can crushed tomatoes

1 (6 ounce) can tomato paste

1 teaspoon salt

1/8 teaspoon pepper

2 Splenda packets

1 cup water

1 bay leaf

2 tablespoons fresh basil (or 2 teaspoons dried, chopped)

Meatloaf

2 lbs ground beef or combination of ground beef, pork and veal

1 cup pork rinds, crushed

2 eggs, beaten

1. Heat oil in skillet on high and sauté mushrooms, onions and garlic. Stir in

tomatoes, tomato paste, salt, pepper and Splenda. Remove and set aside 1- ½ cups of sauce mixture. Add in water, bay leaf and basil. Bring to a boil, reduce heat, cover and simmer for 45 minutes.

2. Combine meat, eggs and pork rinds with reserved herb sauce.
3. Press into loaf or roasting pan and bake at 350 for 45 minutes. Remove loaf from oven, drain and spread 1 cup simmered herb sauce over loaf and return to oven for another 15 minutes.
4. Be sure discard bay leaf before serving. Use remaining her sauce to top off.
5. Yields 8 to 10 servings

[Total Net carbs: 4 grams per serving]

[Total Net carbs for Day 24 based on a single serving per meal: 13 grams]

Day 25

Breakfast Zucchini Muffins

Ingridients

1 cup Atkins Bake Mix

1 cup finely ground almonds

1- ½ cups granular sugar substitute

2 Teaspoons cinnamon

1 Teaspoon salt

1 Teaspoon baking soda

1 Teaspoon baking powder

1 cup canola oil

4 eggs

1 medium zucchini, coarsely grated

1 Teaspoon vanilla extract

1. Preheat oven to 350. Whisk together all dry ingredients in a large bowl. Mix wet ingredients, including zucchini together in a medium bowl. Stir wet ingredients into dry mix slowly, blending well.
2. Pour mixture into a greased 8 x 4 loaf pan or greased muffin tins, depending on your preference. Bake for approximately one hour

until golden brown and toothpick comes out clean.
3. Yields about 12 servings

[Total Net carbs: 3.5 grams per serving]

Lunch

Tuna and Avocado Salad

Ingridients

2 large hard boiled eggs

2 Teaspoons hot sauce

1 cup avocado, mashed

½ cup onion, chopped

1 can tuna

2 Tablespoons mayonnaise

2 Tablespoons pickle relish Fresh lemon juice

Salt, to taste

1. Peel eggs and mince with dinner fork. Peel avocado and squeeze on lemon juice to prevent discoloration. Mash avocado in with egg.
2. Drain tuna and mix into egg/avocado, adding onions, mayonnaise, relish, salt and

hot sauce. Stir well and serve over a bed of fresh lettuce.
3. Yields 4 servings

[Total Net carbs: 9 grams per serving]

Dinner

Dill Trout

Ingridients

2 pounds pan-dressed trout (or other small fish), fresh or frozen

1 ½ Teaspoons salt

¼ Teaspoon pepper

½ cup butter or margarine

2 Tablespoons dill weed

3 Tablespoons lemon juice

1. Cut fish lengthwise and spread open to season with salt and pepper.
2. Prepare a fry pan with melted butter and dill weed. Place fish flesh side down and fry 2-3 minutes per side. Once done, remove fish and add lemon juice to butter and dill to create sauce for garnishing.
3. Yields 6 servings

[Total Net carbs: 1 gram per serving]

[Total Net carbs for Day 25 based on a single serving per meal: 13.5 grams]

Day 26

Breakfast Salmon Omelet

Ingridients

3 eggs

1 smoked salmon

3 links pork sausage

4 onions

1 cup provolone cheese

1. Beat eggs and place into skillet. Follow standard omelet method, adding onions, salmon and cheese before turning omelet over. Sprinkle finished omelet with extra cheese and
2. Serve sausage links on the side.
3. Yields 1 serving

[Total Net carbs: 5.65 grams per serving]

Lunch

Egg Salad over Lettuce

Ingridients

3 eggs

2 Tablespoons mayonnaise

1/8 cup oil roasted sunflower seeds

1 cup shredded lettuce

1. Hard boil eggs and mash together with mayonnaise and sunflower seeds. Spread over shredded lettuce
2. Yields 1 serving

    [Total Net carbs: 5.54 grams per serving]

Dinner

Diet Tuna Casserole

Ingridients

3 hard boiled eggs

1 large can of tuna Mayonnaise to taste

2 cups mild, shredded cheddar cheese

1. Mix mayonnaise and tuna together and spread into small casserole dish. Add a layer of cheese. Slice up boiled eggs and mix with

a little extra mayonnaise and layer them on top of cheese. Add one extra layer of cheese to top off and microwave the casserole until the cheese melts and sizzles.

2. Yields 1 serving

[Total Net carbs: 4 grams per serving]

[Total Net carbs for Day 26 based on a single serving per meal: 15.19 grams]

Day 27

Breakfast

Ingridients

Sausage and Egg Muffins

6 oz Ital. sausage

6 eggs

1/8 cup heavy cream

3 oz cheese

1. Preheat oven to 350 degree. Spray large muffin pans with cooking spray. Cut sausage links and place them 2 to a tin.
2. Mix eggs with cream, salt and pepper. Pour into tins over sausage. Sprinkle with cheese,

layer on remaining egg mixture and top off with cheese again. Bake for approximately 20 minutes or until eggs are done.
3. Yields 3 servings

[Total Net carbs: 2.3 grams per serving]

Lunch

Ham and Cheese Roll

Ingridients

8 ounces cream cheese, softened

2 cup Cheddar cheese, shredded

1 Teaspoon grated onions

1 Teaspoon dry mustard

½ Teaspoon paprika

2 ¼ ounces deviled ham

1 Tablespoon parsley flakes

½ cup pecans, chopped Parsley sprigs

1. Combine all ingredients except parsley and pecans. Mix well and chill for at least one hour. Shape mixture into 8 inch rolls and coat with pecans. Garnish with parsley and serve with crackers.

2. Yields 8 servings

   [*Total Net carbs: 2 grams per serving*]

Dinner

Golden Mushroom Chicken Thighs

Ingridients

5 chicken thighs

1 can golden mushroom soup

1. Remove all skin from thighs and rinse chicken under cold water. Place thighs into a crock pot or slow cooker and pour in mushroom soup. Cook on high for 3-4 hours until meat is tender and fall off the bone.
2. Yields 6 servings

   [*Total Net carbs: 4 grams per serving*]

   [*Total Net carbs for Day 27 based on a single serving per meal: 14.3 grams*]

Day 28

Breakfast

Mexican Breakfast

Ingridients

4 eggs, poached

¼ cup chunky salsa

1/3 cup cheddar cheese, shredded

1/3 cup avocado, cut into chunks

2 Tbs. sour cream

2 Tbs. olives, sliced

2 Tbs. fresh cilantro, finely chopped

1. Cook eggs by poaching method. Heat salsa in microwave or on stove over medium high heat.
2. Place poached eggs on serving plate and top with salsa, sour cream, olives, cheese, avocado and parsley.
3. Yields 2 servings

    [Total Net carbs: 7 grams per serving]

Lunch

Basil Cheese Torta with Red Bell Pepper Strips and Nuts

Ingridients

½ pound cream cheese, softened

4 Tablespoons butter, softened

3/4 cup basil pesto

½ pound Provolone, thinly sliced

¼ cup pine nuts, toasted

1 red bell pepper, roasted, peeled, seeded, and cut into 3" x 3/8" strips 1 small jar sundried tomatoes (packed in olive oil)

Fresh basil for garnish *Requires chilling. Prepare meal in advance so it is ready for Day 28 lunch.

1. Mash cream cheese and butter together with a fork. Add pesto and mix well. Line a bowl with plastic wrap and arrange a think layer of provolone slices.
2. Spread 1/3 pesto over cheese and arrange a few tomatoes, pepper strips and about one Tablespoon pine nuts.
3. Repeat layering until all ingredients are used. Chill overnight.
4. Yields 12 servings

[Total Net carbs: 2 grams per serving]

Dinner

Beef Baked with Yogurt and Black Pepper

Ingridients

6 Tablespoons vegetable oil
2 pounds beef stew meat
3 onions, minced
6 garlic cloves
½ Teaspoon ginger
½ Teaspoon cayenne
1 Tablespoon paprika
2 Teaspoons salt
½ Tablespoon pepper
1 ¼ cups plain yogurt, beaten lightly

1. Preheat oven to 350 Degrees. Heat oil in a large stockpot over medium high heat. Add beef and brown thoroughly. Remove beef when browed and place in a bowl to accumulate juices (juice will be used in recipe).
2. Add onions and garlic to pot and sauté until brown.

3. Return browned meat and juices to pot. Stir in ginger, cayenne, paprika, salt and pepper. Add in yogurt and bring mixture to a simmer. Cover pot with aluminum foil and lid.
4. Place in oven and bake 1 hour. Add water as needed before baking to ensure meat remains tender.
5. Yields 4 to 6 servings

[Total Net carbs: 10 grams per serving]

[Total Net carbs for Day 28 based on a single serving per meal: 19 grams]

Day 29

Breakfast

Orange Nut Muffins

Ingridients

6 eggs, separated

¼ Teaspoon cream of tartar

8 Splenda packets

¼ cup soy flour

¼ cup walnuts, ground

1 Teaspoon orange extract, divided

1 Tablespoon Brown Sugar Twin

4 ounces cream cheese

¼ cup heavy cream

8 Splenda packets

1 Teaspoon orange extract

1. Combine egg whites with cream of tartar and 4 Splenda packets and beat until whites are stiff.
2. Sprinkle on 1 Teaspoon orange extract.
3. In a separate bowl, beat egg yolks together with 4 Splenda packets, and 1 Tablespoon Brown Sugar Twin. Add 1 Teaspoon orange extract. Add a spoonful of egg whites mixture to yolk mixture, stir well, then pour entire yolk mixture into egg whites. Fold in 1 cup soy flour and walnuts.
4. Place mixture into 12 greased muffin cups and bake at 350 for 15 minutes. Reduce oven temperature to 325 and bake for another 15 minutes.
5. Yields 12 servings

    [Total Net carbs: 2.3 grams per serving]

Lunch

German Cucumber Salad

Ingridients
2 cucumbers, thinly sliced
4 green onions, thinly sliced
3 small tomatoes
2 Tablespoons snipped parsley
¼ cup sour cream
¼ Teaspoon mustard
2 Tablespoons minced dill
1 Tablespoon vinegar
1 Tablespoon heavy cream
½ Teaspoon salt
½ Teaspoon pepper

1. Dice and combine cucumbers, onions, tomatoes and parsley. Combine dressing ingredients separately then pour over salad and toss lightly. Chill at least 1 hour before serving.
2. Yields 6 servings

    [Total Net carbs: 9 grams per serving]

Dinner

Turkey Broccoli Casserole

Ingridients

2 (10 ounces) packages frozen broccoli

2 cups cooked and diced turkey

1 (10 ounce) can cream of mushroom soup

½ cup heavy cream

½ cup Cheddar cheese, grated

1. Preheat oven to 375. Cook broccoli according to package directions. Layer broccoli in a baking dish and spread turkey on top.
2. Combine soup with cream and pour on top of turkey. Sprinkle on grated cheese. Place in oven and bake for 30 minutes.
3. Yields 8 servings

   [Total Net carbs: 7 grams per serving]

   [Total Net carbs for Day 29 based on a single serving per meal: 19.3 grams]

Day 30

Breakfast

Cinnamon Bran Muffins

Ingridients

3 eggs, separated
2 Tbs butter, melted
2 Tbs coconut oil, melted
½ cup Designer® Protein (French vanilla)
2 Tbs soy flour
2 Tbs wheat bran, toasted
¼ cup walnuts, toasted
¼ tsp ground cinnamon
1/8 tsp stevia (a non-caloric, natural herbal sweetener, found in health food stores)
2 tsp baking powder

1. Separate eggs and beat egg whites until they form stiff peaks. In a medium bowl, beat egg yolks with butter and coconut oil. In a separate bowl, mix whey protein, soy flour, wheat bran, walnuts, cinnamon, stevia and baking powder. Beat dry mixture into egg yolk combination.

Gently fold egg whites into batter and pour into a buttered nonstick muffin pan.
2. Bake in a preheated oven at 350 Degree for 30 minutes, or until inserted toothpick comes out clean.
3. Yields 8 servings

[Total Net carbs: 3 grams per serving]

Lunch

Sausage Frittata

Ingridients

8 ounces sausage

½ onion, chopped

2 garlic clove, minced

½ cup ricotta

½ cup heavy cream

4 eggs

¼ Teaspoon cayenne

¼ cup salsa

1 cup Cheddar cheese, shredded

Salt to taste

1. Preheat oven to 350 Degree. Sauté onion and garlic in skillet, then add sausage and brown,

mincing as it cooks. In a mixing bowl, beat eggs, cream and seasoning in a bowl.
2. Add salsa. Pour mixture over sausage. Place skillet in oven and bake until eggs are set. Top with cheese and heat under broiler until melted.
3. Yields 4 servings

[Total Net carbs: 6 grams per serving]

Dinner

Deviled Chicken Halves

Ingridients

1 chicken

¼ cup butter

2 Tablespoons lemon juice

2 Tablespoons vegetable oil

1 Teaspoon mustard

¼ Teaspoon cayenne

¼ cup minced green onion

1 Teaspoon minced garlic

1. Preheat broiler. Wash chicken and split down the middle into halves. Combine butter, oil,

mustard, cayenne and lemon juice in a small mixing bowl. Brush chicken with mixture. Next, add onions, garlic and salt into remaining mixture.
2. Place chicken in a broiler pan, skin side down. Broil for 20 minutes, then turn and broil other side for 10 minutes. Baste with remaining butter mixture and broil another 10 minutes until chicken is tender.
3. Serve with lemon wedges.
4. Yields 4 servings

[Total Net carbs: 2 grams per serving]

[Total Net carbs for Day 30 based on a single serving per meal: 11 grams]

Conclusion

I hope you have found this book in good health, and I wish you continued success on your low carb diet. Whenever you find yourself retreating back to the old unhealthy lifestyle, please refer back to this book, it will get you back on the path to success.

This is my small contribution to the worldwide phenomenon knows as the Low Carb Diet, and my hope is only to be able to help one person in need. Should I meet that goal, and you feel you have benefited from reading and using these principles, please feel free to drop me a line of review and let me know what you think about this book. I will be eternally grateful.

After you have completed the 30-day cycle, your work is not complete. Always remember, 'weight is managed, not cured'. After you have been on a low carb diet for any time, you will begin to notice the approximate place you should be at in your daily 'net carbs' to easily be able to maintain your weight loss for life.

I highly recommend that you keep accurate data on your daily food consumption, and I honestly do not know of an easier way to do this, than cooking from the cookbook.

Kitchen Measurements

US Dry Volume Measurements

1/16 tea spoon – dash

1/8 tea spoon – a pinch

3 (three) tea spoons – 1(one) table spoon

1/8 cup – 2 (two) table spoons

¼ (one-quarter) cup – 4 (four) table spoons

1/3 (one-third) cup – 5 (five) table spoons + 1 (one) tea spoon

½ (half) cup – 8 (eight) table spoons

¾ (three-quarter) cup – 12 (twelve) table spoons

1 (one) cup – 16 (sixteen) table spoons

1 (one) pound – 16 (sixteen) ounces

US Liquid Measurements

8 (eight) fluid ounces – 1 (one) cup

1 (one) pint – 2 (two) cups (16 fluid ounces)

1 (one) quart – 2 (two) pints (4 cups)

1 (one) Gallon – 4 quarts (16 cups)

Metric to US Conversation

1 (one) milliliter – 1/5 teaspoon

5ml – 1 (one) teaspoon

15 ml – 1 (one) tablespoon

30ml – 1 fluid oz

100ml – 3.4fluid oz

240ml – 1 (one) cup

1 (one) liter – 34 fluid oz

1 (one) liter – 4.2 cups

1 liter – 2.1 pints

1 liter – 1.06 quarts

1 liter - .26 gallon

1 gram - .035 ounces

100gram – 3.5 ounces

500 gram – 1.10 pounds

1kilogram – 2.205 pounds

1 kilogram – 35oz

Made in the USA
Columbia, SC
08 March 2018